Alkaline Smoothies

A Complete Collection of Clean and Innovative Smoothies

Isaac Vinson

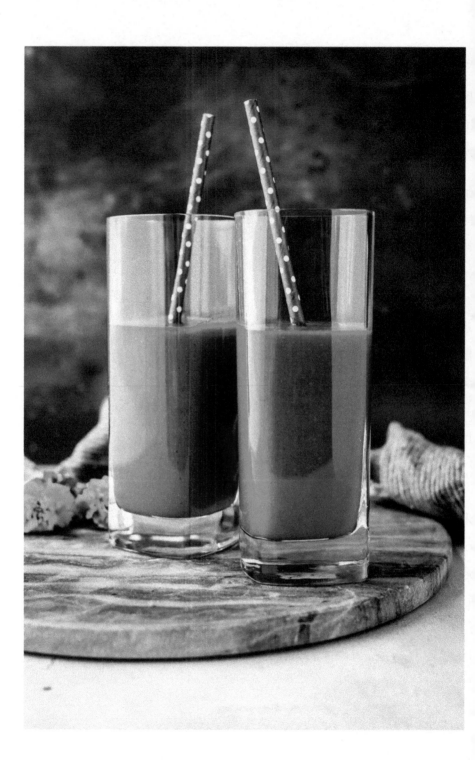

Table of Contents

RED VEGGIE & FRUIT SMOOTHIE 6

KALE SMOOTHIE.. 8

GREEN TOFU SMOOTHIE 10

GRAPE & SWISS CHARD SMOOTHIE 13

MATCHA CREAMED SMOOTHIE.. 15

BANANA SMOOTHIE.. 18

STRAWBERRY CREAMED SMOOTHIE 20

RASPBERRY & TOFU SMOOTHIE...23

MANGO SMOOTHIE...26

PINEAPPLE SMOOTHIE...28

KALE & PINEAPPLE SMOOTHIE..30

GREEN VEGGIES SMOOTHIE 33

AVOCADO & SPINACH SMOOTHIE..36

DANDELION AVOCADO SMOOTHIE..38

AMARANTH GREENS AND AVOCADO SMOOTHIE 40

LETTUCE, ORANGE AND BANANA SMOOTHIE..42

DELICIOUS ELDERBERRY SMOOTHIE 44

PEACHES ZUCCHINI SMOOTHIE 45

GINGER ORANGE AND STRAWBERRY SMOOTHIE 48

KALE PARSLEY AND CHIA SEEDS DETOX SMOOTHIE.......................................50

WATERMELON LIMENADE 52

BUBBLY ORANGE SODA...54

CREAMY CASHEW MILK...56

HOMEMADE OAT MILK..58

LUCKY MINT SMOOTHIE..60

PARADISE ISLAND SMOOTHIE 62

APPLE PIE SMOOTHIE...64

DETOX APPLE SMOOTHIE 67

BERRIES AND HEMP SEEDS SMOOTHIE 69

PEAR, BERRIES, AND QUINOA SMOOTHIE..71

MANGO AND BANANA SMOOTHIE...73

BERRIES AND SEA MOSS SMOOTHIE 75

RASPBERRY AND CHARD SMOOTHIE 77

APPLE, BERRIES, AND KALE SMOOTHIE..80

BANANA, BERRY, AND KALE SMOOTHIE...82

BANANA AND FLAX SMOOTHIE 84

APPLE JUICE MIX 86

STOMACH SOOTHER..89

SARSAPARILLA SYRUP 91

DANDELION "COFFEE"...93

CHAMOMILE DELIGHT 95

CLEANSE TEA...97

IMMUNE TEA 100

GINGER TURMERIC TEA...102

RELAX TEA 104

Red Veggie & Fruit Smoothie

Preparation Time: 10 minutes

Cooking Time: 0 minutes

Servings: 2

Ingredients :

• ½ cup fresh raspberries

• ½ cup fresh strawberries

• ½ red bell pepper, seeded and chopped

• ½ cup red cabbage, chopped

• 1 small tomato

• 1 cup water

• ½ cup ice cubes

Directions:

1. Place all the Ingredients in a high-speed blender and pulse until creamy.

2. Pour the smoothie into two glasses and serve immediately.

Nutrition:

Calories 39

Cholesterol 0 mg

Saturated Fat 0 g

Sodium 10 mg

Total Carbs 8.9 g

Fiber 3.5 g

Sugar 4.8 g

Protein 1.3 g

Total Fat 0.4 g

Kale Smoothie

Preparation Time: 10 minutes

Cooking Time: 0 minutes

Servings: 2

Ingredients :

3 stalks fresh kale, trimmed and chopped

1-2 celery stalks, chopped

½ avocado, peeled, pitted, and chopped

½-inch piece ginger root, chopped

½-inch piece turmeric root, chopped

2 cups coconut milk

Directions:

1. Place all the Ingredients in a high-speed blender and pulse until creamy.

2. Pour the smoothie into two glasses and serve immediately.

Nutrition:

Calories 248

Total Fat 22.8 g

Saturated Fat 12 g

Cholesterol 0 mg

Sodium 59 mg

Total Carbs 11.3 g

Fiber 4.2 g

Sugar 0.5 g

Protein 3.5 g

Green Tofu Smoothie

Preparation Time: 10 minutes
Cooking Time: 0 minutes
Servings: 2

Ingredients :

• 1½ cups cucumber, peeled and chopped roughly

• 3 cups fresh baby spinach

• 2 cups frozen broccoli

• ½ cup silken tofu, drained and pressed

• 1 tablespoon fresh lime juice

• 4-5 drops liquid stevia

• 1 cup unsweetened almond milk

• ½ cup ice, crushed

Directions:

1. Place all the Ingredients in a high-speed blender and pulse until creamy.

2. Pour the smoothie into two glasses and serve immediately.

Nutrition:

Calories 118

Total Fat 15 g

Saturated Fat 0.8 g

Cholesterol 0 mg

Sodium 165 mg

Total Carbs 12.6 g

Fiber 4.8 g

Sugar 3.4 g

Protein 10 g

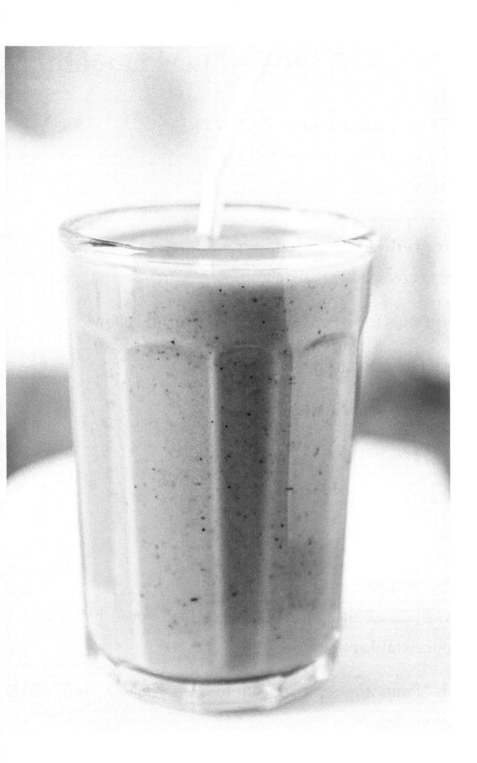

Grape & Swiss Chard Smoothie

Preparation Time: 10 minutes

Cooking Time: 0 minutes

Servings: 2

Ingredients :

- 2 cups seedless green grapes

- 2 cups fresh Swiss chard, trimmed and chopped

- 2 tablespoons maple syrup

- 1 teaspoon fresh lemon juice

- 1½ cups water

- 4 ice cubes

Directions:

1. Place all the Ingredients in a high-speed blender and pulse until creamy.

2. Pour the smoothie into two glasses and serve immediately.

Nutrition:

Calories 176

Total Fat 0.2 g

Saturated Fat 0 g

Cholesterol 0 mg

Sodium 83 mg

Total Carbs 44.9 g

Fiber 1.7 g

Sugar 37.9 g

Protein 0.7 g

Matcha Creamed Smoothie

Preparation Time: 10 minutes
Cooking Time: 0 minutes
Servings: 2

Ingredients :

• 2 tablespoons chia seeds

• 2 teaspoons matcha green tea powder

• ½ teaspoon fresh lemon juice

• ½ teaspoon xanthan gum

• 8-10 drops liquid stevia

• 4 tablespoons coconut cream

• 1½ cups unsweetened almond milk

• ¼ cup ice cubes

Directions:

1. Place all the Ingredients in a high-speed blender and pulse until creamy.

2. Pour the smoothie into two glasses and serve immediately.

Nutrition:

Calories 132

Total Fat 12.3 g

Saturated Fat 6.8 g

Cholesterol 0 mg

Sodium 15 mg

Total Carbs 7 g

Fiber 4.8 g

Sugar 1 g

Protein 3 g

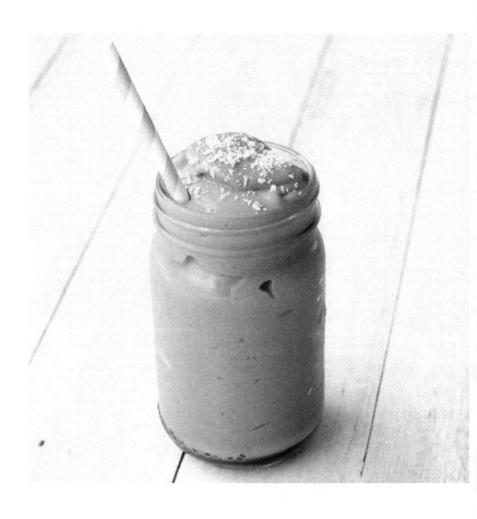

Banana Smoothie

Preparation Time: 10 minutes

Cooking Time: 0 minutes

Servings: 2

Ingredients :

• 2 cups chilled unsweetened almond milk

• 1 large frozen banana, peeled and sliced

• 1 tablespoon almonds, chopped

• 1 teaspoon organic vanilla extract

Directions:

1. Place all the Ingredients in a high-speed blender and pulse until creamy.

2. Pour the smoothie into two glasses and serve immediately.

Nutrition:

Calories 124

Total Fat 5.2 g

Saturated Fat 0.5 g

Cholesterol 0 mg

Sodium 181 mg

Total Carbs 18.4 g

Fiber 3.1 g

Sugar 8.7 g

Protein 2.4 g

Strawberry Creamed Smoothie

Preparation Time: 10 minutes
Cooking Time: 0 minutes
Servings: 2

Ingredients :

2 cups chilled unsweetened almond milk

1½ cups frozen strawberries

1 banana, peeled and sliced

¼ teaspoon organic vanilla extract

Directions:

. Add all the Ingredients in a high-speed blender and pulse until smooth.

. Pour the smoothie into two glasses and serve immediately.

Nutrition:

Calories 131

Total Fat 3.7 g

Saturated Fat 0.4 g

Cholesterol 0 mg

Sodium 181 mg

Total Carbs 25.3 g

Fiber 4.8 g

Sugar 14 g

Protein 1.6 g

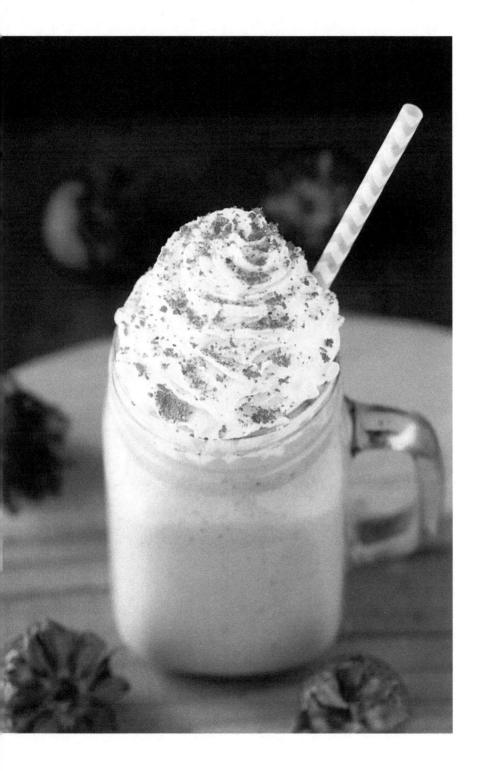

Raspberry & Tofu Smoothie

Preparation Time: 15 minutes
Cooking Time: 0 minutes
Servings: 2

Ingredients :

• 1½ cups fresh raspberries

• 6 ounces firm silken tofu, drained

• 1/8 teaspoon coconut extract

• 1 teaspoon powdered stevia

• 1½ cups unsweetened almond milk

• ¼ cup ice cubes, crushed

Directions:

1. Add all the Ingredients in a high-speed blender and pulse until smooth.

2. Pour the smoothie into two glasses and serve immediately.

Nutrition:

Calories 131

Total Fat 5.5 g

Saturated Fat 0.6 g

Cholesterol 0 mg

Sodium 167 mg

Total Carbs 14.6 g

Fiber 6.8 g

Sugar 5.2 g

Protein 7.7 g

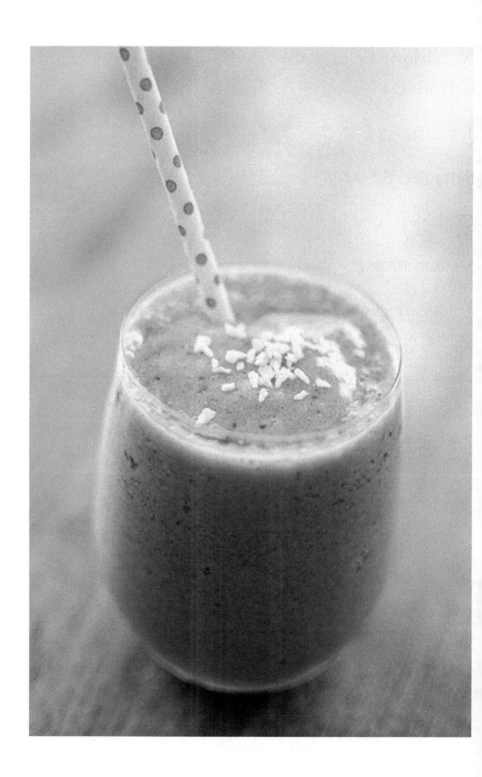

Mango Smoothie

Preparation Time: 10 minutes

Cooking Time: 0 minutes

Servings: 2

Ingredients :

2 cups frozen mango, peeled, pitted and chopped

¼ cup almond butter

Pinch of ground turmeric

2 tablespoons fresh lemon juice

1¼ cups unsweetened almond milk

¼ cup ice cubes

Directions:

1. Add all the Ingredients in a high-speed blender and pulse until smooth.

2. Pour the smoothie into two glasses and serve immediately.

Nutrition:

Calories 140

Total Fat 4.1 g

Saturated Fat 0.6 g

Cholesterol 0 mg

Sodium 118 mg

Total Carbs 26.8 g

Fiber 3.6 g

Sugar 23 g

Protein 2.5 g

Pineapple Smoothie

Preparation Time: 10 minutes

Cooking Time: 0 minutes

Servings: 2

Ingredients :

• 2 cups pineapple, chopped

• ½ teaspoon fresh ginger, peeled and chopped

• ½ teaspoon ground turmeric

• 1 teaspoon natural immune support supplement *

• 1 teaspoon chia seeds

• 1½ cups cold green tea

• ½ cup ice, crushed

Directions:

1. Add all the Ingredients in a high-speed blender and pulse until smooth.

2. Pour the smoothie into two glasses and serve immediately.

Nutrition:

Calories 152

Total Fat 1 g

Saturated Fat 0 g

Cholesterol 0 mg

Sodium 9 mg

Total Carbs 30 g

Fiber 3.5 g

Sugar 29.8 g

Protein 1.5 g

Kale & Pineapple Smoothie

Preparation Time: 15 minutes

Cooking Time: 0 minutes

Servings: 2

Ingredients :

• 1½ cups fresh kale, trimmed and chopped

• 1 frozen banana, peeled and chopped

• ½ cup fresh pineapple chunks

• 1 cup unsweetened coconut milk

• ½ cup fresh orange juice

• ½ cup ice

Directions:

1. Add all the Ingredients in a high-speed blender and pulse until smooth.

2. Pour the smoothie into two glasses and serve immediately.

Nutrition:

Calories 148

Total Fat 2.4 g

Saturated Fat 2.1 g

Cholesterol 0 mg

Sodium 23 mg

Total Carbs 31.6 g

Fiber 3.5 g

Sugar 16.5 g

Protein 2.8 g

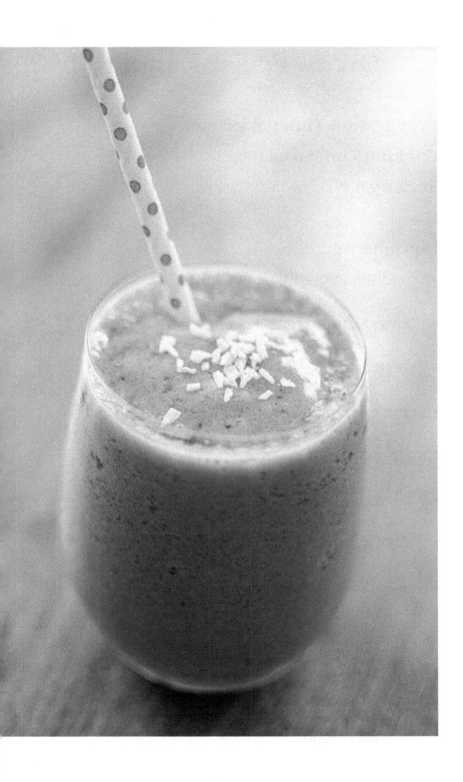

Green Veggies Smoothie

Preparation Time: 15 minutes

Cooking Time: 0 minutes

Servings: 2

Ingredients :

• 1 medium avocado, peeled, pitted, and chopped

• 1 large cucumber, peeled and chopped

• 2 fresh tomatoes, chopped

• 1 small green bell pepper, seeded and chopped

• 1 cup fresh spinach, torn

• 2 tablespoons fresh lime juice

• 2 tablespoons homemade vegetable broth

• 1 cup alkaline water

Directions:

1. Add all the Ingredients in a high-speed blender and pulse until smooth.

2. Pour the smoothie into glasses and serve immediately.

Nutrition:

Calories 275

Total Fat 20.3 g

Saturated Fat 4.2 g

Cholesterol 0 mg

Sodium 76 mg

Total Carbs 24.1 g

Fiber 10.1 g

Sugar 9.3 g

Protein 5.3 g

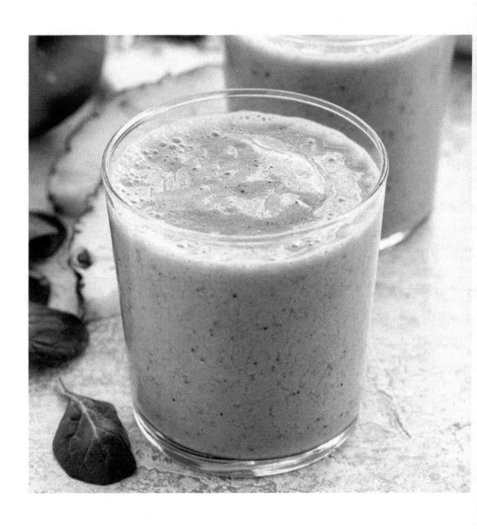

Avocado & Spinach Smoothie

Preparation Time: 10 minutes
Cooking Time: 0 minutes
Servings: 2

Ingredients :

• 2 cups fresh baby spinach

• ½ avocado, peeled, pitted, and chopped

• 4-6 drops liquid stevia

• ½ teaspoon ground cinnamon

• 1 tablespoon hemp seeds

• 2 cups chilled alkaline water

Directions:

1. Add all the Ingredients in a high-speed blender and pulse until smooth.

2. Pour the smoothie into two glasses and serve immediately.

Nutrition:

Calories 132

Total Fat 11.7 g

Saturated Fat 2.2 g

Cholesterol 0 mg

Sodium 27 mg

Total Carbs 6.1 g

Fiber 4.5 g

Sugar 0.4 g

Protein 3.1 g

Dandelion Avocado Smoothie

Preparation Time: 15 minutes

Cooking Time: 0

Servings: 1

Ingredients :

One cup of Dandelion

One Orange (juiced)

Coconut water

One Avocado

One key lime (juice)

Directions:

1. In a high-speed blender until smooth, blend ingredients

Nutrition:

Calories: 160

Fat: 15 grams

Carbohydrates: 9 grams

Protein: 2 grams

Amaranth Greens And Avocado Smoothie

Preparation Time: 15 minutes

Cooking Time: 0

Servings: 1

Ingredients :

• One key lime (juice).

• Two sliced apples (seeded).

• Half avocado.

• Two cupsful of amaranth greens.

• Two cupsful of watercress.

• One cupful of water.

Directions:

Add the whole recipes together and transfer them into the blender. Blend thoroughly until smooth.

Nutrition:

Calories: 160

Fat: 15 grams

Carbohydrates: 9 grams

Protein: 2 grams

Lettuce, Orange And Banana Smoothie

Preparation Time: 15 minutes

Cooking Time: 0

Servings: 1

Ingredients :

• One and a half cupsful of fresh lettuce.

• One large banana.

• One cup of mixed berries of your choice.

• One juiced orange.

Directions:

1. First, add the orange juice to your blender.

2. Add the remaining recipes and blend thoroughly.

3. Enjoy the rest of your day.

Nutrition:

Calories: 252.1

Protein: 4.1 g

Delicious Elderberry Smoothie

Preparation Time: 15 minutes

Cooking Time: 0

Servings: 1

Ingredients :

One cupful of Elderberry

One cupful of Cucumber

One large apple

A quarter cupful of water

Directions:

Add the whole recipes together into a blender. Grind very well until they are uniformly smooth and enjoy.

Nutrition:

Calories: 106

Carbohydrates: 26.68

Peaches Zucchini Smoothie

Preparation Time: 15 minutes

Cooking Time: 0

Servings: 1

Ingredients :

• A half cupful of squash.

• A half cupful of peaches.

• A quarter cupful of coconut water.

• A half cupful of Zucchini.

Directions:

1. Add the whole recipes together into a blender and blend until smooth and serve.

Nutrition:

55 Calories

0g Fat

2g Of Protein

10mg Sodium

14 G Carbohydrate

2g Of Fiber

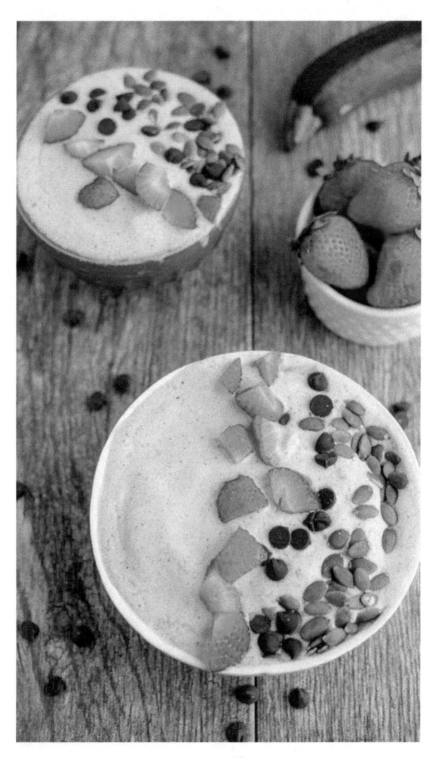

Ginger Orange And Strawberry Smoothie

Preparation Time: 15 minutes

Cooking Time: 0

Servings: 1

Ingredients :

• One cup of strawberry.

• One large orange (juice)

• One large banana.

• Quarter small sized ginger (peeled and sliced).

Directions:

2. Transfer the orange juice to a clean blender.

3. Add the remaining recipes and blend thoroughly until smooth.

4. Enjoy. Wow! You have ended the 9th day of your weight loss and detox journey.

Nutrition:

32 Calories

0.3g Fat

2g Of Protein

10mg Sodium

14g Carbohydrate

Water

2g Of Fiber.

Kale Parsley And Chia Seeds Detox Smoothie

Preparation Time: 15 minutes

Cooking Time: 0

Servings: 1

Ingredients :

• Three tbsp. chia seeds (grounded).

• One cupful of water.

• One sliced banana.

• One pear (chopped).

• One cupful of organic kale.

• One cupful of parsley.

• Two tbsp. of lemon juice.

• A dash of cinnamon.

Directions:

Add the whole recipes together into a blender and pour the water before blending. Blend at high speed until smooth and enjoy. You may or may not place it in the refrigerator depending on how hot or cold the weather appears.

Nutrition:

75 calories

1g fat

5g protein

10g fibre

Watermelon Limenade

Preparation Time: 5 Minutes

Cooking Time: 0 minutes

Servings: 6

When it comes to refreshing summertime drinks, lemonade is always near the top of the list. This Watermelon "Limenade" is perfect for using up leftover watermelon or for those early fall days when stores and farmers are almost giving them away. You can also substitute 4 cups of ice for the cold water to create a delicious summertime slushy.

Ingredients

• 4 cups diced watermelon

• 4 cups cold water

• 2 tablespoons freshly squeezed lemon juice

• 1 tablespoon freshly squeezed lime juice

Directions:

1. In a blender, combine the watermelon, water, lemon juice, and lime juice, and blend for 1 minute.

2. Strain the contents through a fine-mesh sieve or nut-milk bag. Serve chilled. Store in the refrigerator for up to 3 days.

SERVING TIP: Slice up a few lemon or lime wedges to serve with your Watermelon Limenade, or top it with a few fresh mint leaves to give it an extra-crisp, minty flavor.

Nutrition:

Calories: 60

Bubbly Orange Soda

Preparation Time: 5 Minutes

Cooking Time: 0 minutes

Servings: 4

Soda can be one of the toughest things to give up when you first adopt a WFPB diet. That's partially because refined sugars and caffeine are addictive, but it can also be because carbonated beverages are fun to drink! With sweetness from the orange juice and bubbliness from the carbonated water, this orange "soda" is perfect for assisting in the transition from SAD to WFPB.

Ingredients

• 4 cups carbonated water

• 2 cups pulp-free orange juice (4 oranges, freshly squeezed and strained)

Directions:

1. For each serving, pour 2 parts carbonated water and 1-part orange juice over ice right before serving.

2. Stir and enjoy.

SERVING TIP: This recipe is best made right before drinking. The amount of fizz in the carbonated water will decrease the longer it's open, so if you're going to make it ahead of time, make sure it's stored in an airtight, refrigerator-safe container.

Nutrition:

Calories: 56

Creamy Cashew Milk

Preparation Time: 5 Minutes

Cooking Time: 0 minutes

Servings: 8

Learning how to make your own plant-based milks can be one of the best ways to save money and ditch dairy for good. This is one of the easiest milk recipes to master, and if you have a high-speed blender, you can skip the straining step and go straight to a refrigerator-safe container. Large mason jars work great for storing plant-based milk, as they allow you to give a quick shake before each use.

Ingredients

4 cups water

¼ cup raw cashews, soaked overnight

Directions:

. In a blender, blend the water and cashews on high speed for 2 minutes.

2. Strain with a nut-milk bag or cheesecloth, then store in the refrigerator for up to 5 days.

VARIATION TIP: This recipe makes unsweetened cashew milk that can be used in savory and sweet dishes. For a creamier version to put in your coffee, cut the amount of water in half. For a sweeter version, add 1 to 2 tablespoons maple syrup and 1 teaspoon vanilla extract before blending.

Nutrition:

Calories: 18

Homemade Oat Milk

Preparation Time: 5 Minutes

Cooking Time: 0 minutes

Servings: 8

Oat milk is a fantastic option if you need a nut-free milk or just want an extremely inexpensive plant-based milk. Making a half-gallon jar at home costs a fraction of the price of other plant-based or dairy milks. Oat milk can be used in both savory and sweet dishes.

Ingredients

• 1 cup rolled oats

• 4 cups water

Directions:

1. Put the oats in a medium bowl, and cover with cold water. Soak for 15 minutes, then drain and rinse the oats.

2. Pour the cold water and the soaked oats into a blender. Blend for 60 to 90 seconds, or just until the mixture is a creamy white color throughout. (Blending any further may overblend the oats, resulting in a gummy milk.)

3. Strain through a nut-milk bag or colander, then store in the refrigerator for up to 5 days.

VARIATION TIP: This recipe can easily be made into chocolate oat milk. Once you've strained the oat milk, return it to a blender with 3 tablespoons cocoa powder, 2 tablespoons maple syrup, and 1 teaspoon vanilla extract, then blend for 30 seconds.

Nutrition:

Calories: 39

Lucky Mint Smoothie

Preparation Time: 5 Minutes

Cooking Time: 0 minutes

Servings: 2

As spring approaches and mint begins to once again take over the garden, "Irish"-themed green shakes begin to pop up as well. In contrast to the traditionally high-fat, sugary shakes, this smoothie is a wonderful option for sunny spring days. So next time you want to sip on something cool and minty, do so with a health-promoting Lucky Mint Smoothie.

Ingredients

• 2 cups plant-based milk (here or here)

• 2 frozen bananas, halved

• 1 tablespoon fresh mint leaves or ¼ teaspoon peppermint extract

• 1 teaspoon vanilla extract

Directions:

1. In a blender, combine the milk, bananas, mint, and vanilla. Blend on high for 1 to 2 minutes, or until the contents reach a smooth and creamy consistency, and serve.

VARIATION TIP: If you like to sneak greens into smoothies, add a cup or two of spinach to boost the health benefits of this smoothie and give it an even greener appearance.

Nutrition:

Calories: 152

Paradise Island Smoothie

Preparation Time: 5 Minutes
Cooking Time: 0 minutes
Servings: 2

Ingredients :

  2 cups plant-based milk (here or here)

  1 frozen banana

  ½ cup frozen mango chunks

  ½ cup frozen pineapple chunks

  1 teaspoon vanilla extract

Directions:

1. In a blender, combine the milk, banana, mango, pineapple, and vanilla. Blend on high for 1 to 2 minutes, or until the contents reach a smooth and creamy consistency, and serve.

LEFTOVER TIP: If you have any leftover smoothie, you can put it in a jar with some rolled oats and allow the mixture to soak in the refrigerator overnight to create a tropical version of overnight oats.

Nutrition:

Calories: 176

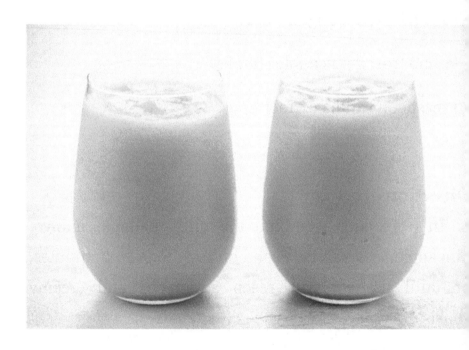

Apple Pie Smoothie

Preparation Time: 5 Minutes

Cooking Time: 0 minutes

Servings: 2

This smoothie is great for a quick breakfast or a cool dessert. Its combination of sweet apples and warming cinnamon is sure to win over children and adults alike. If the holidays find you in a warm area, this smoothie may just be the cool treat you've been looking for to take the place of pie at dessert time.

Ingredients

• 2 sweet crisp apples, cut into 1-inch cubes

• 2 cups plant-based milk (here or here)

• 1 cup ice

• 1 tablespoon maple syrup

• 1 teaspoon ground cinnamon

• 1 teaspoon vanilla extract

Directions:

1. In a blender, combine the apples, milk, ice, maple syrup, cinnamon, and vanilla. Blend on high for 1 to 2 minutes, or until the contents reach a smooth and creamy consistency, and serve.

VARIATION TIP: You can also use this recipe for making overnight oatmeal. Blend your smoothie, mix it with 2 cups rolled oats, and refrigerate overnight for a premade breakfast for two.

Nutrition:

Calories: 198

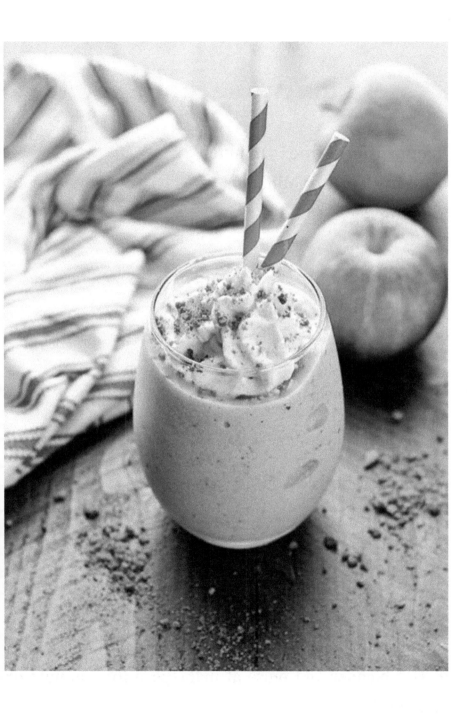

Detox Apple Smoothie

Preparation Time: 5 minutes

Cooking Time: 0 Minutes

Servings: 2

Ingredients

• 2 cups spring water

• 2 cups amaranth greens

• 2 medium fresh apples, cored

• 1 key lime, juiced

• ¼ of avocado

Directions:

1. Take a high-powered blender, switch it on, and then place all the Ingredients inside.

2. Use blender and pulse at high speed for 1 minute or more until

Nutrition:

Calories – 141

Carbohydrates – 27.5 g

Fat – 2.8 g

Fiber – 7.5 g

Protein – 1.4 g

Sugar – 20.1 g

Berries And Hemp Seeds Smoothie

Preparation Time: 5 minutes

Cooking Time: 0 Minutes

Servings: 2

Ingredients

• 1 cup spring water

• 2 cups fresh lettuce

• 1 medium banana, peeled

• 1 cup mixed berries, fresh

• 1 Seville orange, peeled

• 1 tablespoon hemp seeds

• ¼ of avocado pitted

Directions:

1. Take a high-powered blender, switch it on, and then place all the Ingredients inside.

2. Use blender and pulse at high speed for 1 minute or more

Nutrition:

Calories – 216

Carbohydrates – 36.2 g

Fat – 5.5 g

Fiber – 10.8 g

Protein – 5.4 g

Sugar – 23.2 g

Pear, Berries, And Quinoa Smoothie

Preparation Time: 5 minutes

Cooking Time: 0 Minutes

Servings: 2

Ingredients

• 2 cups spring water

• ½ of avocado pitted

• 2 fresh pears, chopped

• ½ cup cooked quinoa

• ¼ cup fresh whole blueberries

Directions:

1. Take a high-powered blender, switch it on, and then place all the Ingredients inside.

2. Use blender and pulse at high speed for 1 minute or more

Nutrition:

Calories – 325.5

Carbohydrates – 57 g

Fat – 7.6 g

Fiber – 11.4 g

Protein – 7.3 g

Sugar – 22 g

Mango And Banana Smoothie

Preparation Time: 5 minutes

Cooking Time: 0 Minutes

Servings: 2

Ingredients

• 1 cup spring water

• 2 cups greens

• ½ of banana, peeled

• 1 fresh mango, peeled, destoned, sliced

Directions:

1. Take a high-powered blender, switch it on, and then place all the Ingredients inside.

2. Use blender and pulse at high speed for 1 minute or more

Nutrition:

Calories – 134.5

Carbohydrates – 29.6 g

Fat – 1 g

Fiber – 4.3 g

Protein – 1.7 g

Sugar – 26.8

Berries And Sea Moss Smoothie

Preparation Time: 5 minutes

Cooking Time: 0 Minutes

Servings: 2

Ingredients

• 1 cup of coconut water

• 2 cups lettuce leaves

• 1 banana, peeled

• 1 cup mixed berries

• 1 tablespoon sea moss

• 2 key limes, juiced

Directions:

1. Take a high-powered blender, switch it on, and then place all the Ingredients inside.

2. Use blender and pulse at high speed for 1 minute or more

Nutrition:

Calories – 163

Carbohydrates – 35 g

Fat – 0.9 g

Fiber – 10 g

Protein – 3.7 g

Sugar – 20.7 g

Raspberry And Chard Smoothie

Preparation Time: 5 minutes

Cooking Time: 0 Minutes

Servings: 2

Ingredients

• 2 cups of coconut water

• 2 cups Swiss chards

• 2 key limes, juiced

• 2 cups fresh whole raspberries

Directions:

1. Take a high-powered blender, switch it on, and then place all the Ingredients inside.

2. Use blender and pulse at high speed for 1 minute or more

Nutrition:

Calories – 137.5

Carbohydrates – 27.8 g

Fat – 1.4 g

Fiber – 13.2 g

Protein – 3.4 g

Sugar – 13.4 g

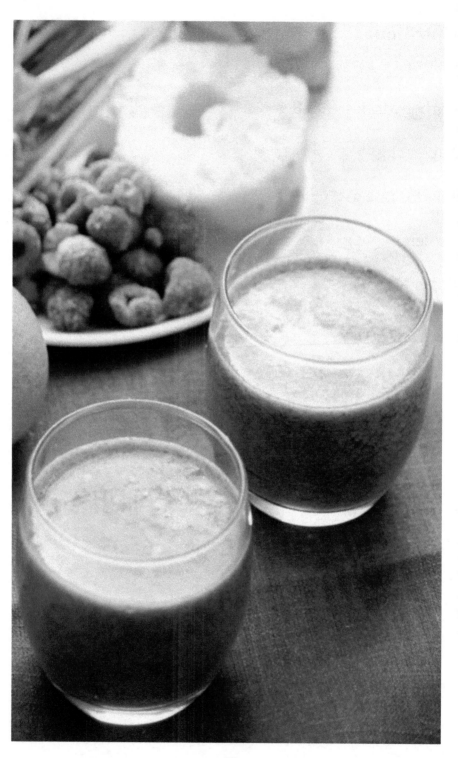

Apple, Berries, And Kale Smoothie

Preparation Time: 5 minutes

Cooking Time: 0 Minutes

Servings: 2

Ingredients

1 cup spring water

1 cup mixed berries

2 cups kale leaves, fresh

1 large apple, cored

Directions:

1. Take a high-powered blender, switch it on, and then place all the Ingredients inside.

2. Use blender and pulse at high speed for 1 minute or more

Nutrition:

Calories – 112

Carbohydrates – 24.4 g

Fat – 0.7 g

Fiber – 7.2 g

Protein – 2 g

Sugar – 18.3 g

Banana, Berry, And Kale Smoothie

Preparation Time: 5 minutes

Cooking Time: 0 Minutes

Servings: 2

Ingredients

• 2 cups fresh whole strawberries

• 2 bananas, peeled

• 2 cups chopped kale

• 1 cup of ice cubes

Directions:

1. Take a high-powered blender, switch it on, and then place all the Ingredients inside.

2. Use blender and pulse at high speed for 1 minute or more

Nutrition:

Calories – 185

Carbohydrates – 40.7 g

Fat – 1.2 g

Fiber – 8.5 g

Protein – 2.8 g

Sugar – 25.8 g

Banana And Flax Smoothie

Preparation Time: 5 minutes

Cooking Time: 0 Minutes

Servings: 2

Ingredients

• 1 cup spring water

• 2 cups spinach, fresh

• 1 banana, peeled

• ½ cup fresh whole blueberries

• 1 tablespoon flax seeds

Directions:

1. Take a high-powered blender, switch it on, and then place all the Ingredients inside.

2. Use blender and pulse at high speed for 1 minute or more

Nutrition:

Calories – 107.5

Carbohydrates – 20.4 g

Fat – 2 g

Fiber – 4.7 g

Protein – 1.9 g

Sugar – 12.3 g

Apple Juice Mix

Preparation Time: 5 minutes
Cooking Time: 0 Minutes
Servings: 2

Ingredients

1 1/2 cups apple juice, fresh

1 medium apple, peeled, cored

2 cups kale leaves, fresh

½ of avocado pitted

Directions:

1. Take a high-powered blender, switch it on, and then place all the Ingredients inside.

2. Use blender and pulse at high speed for 1 minute or more

Nutrition:

Calories – 197

Carbohydrates – 35.5 g

Fat – 5.5 g

Fiber – 5.8 g

Protein – 1.5 g

Sugar – 27.7 g

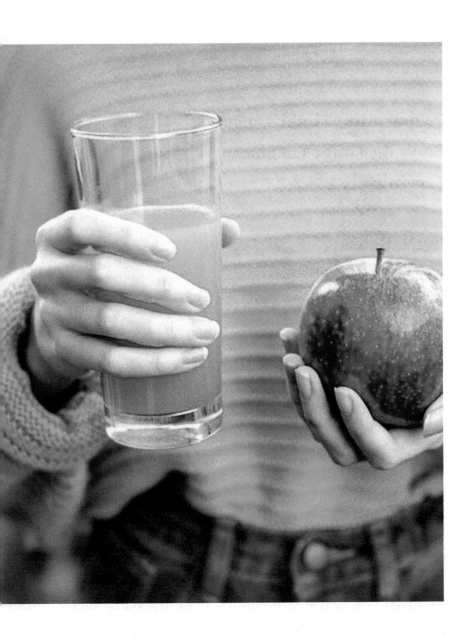

Stomach Soother

Preparation Time: 5 minutes

Cooking Time: 3 minutes

Servings: 1

Ingredients :

• Agave syrup, 1 tbsp.

• Ginger tea, .5 c

• Alkaline Stomach Relief Herbal Tea

• Burro banana, 1

Directions:

1. Fix the herbal tea according to the Directions on the package. Set it aside to cool.

2. Once the tea is cool, place it along with all the other Ingredients into a blender. Switch on the blender and let it run until it is creamy.

Nutrition:

Calories 25

Sugar 3g

Protein 0.3g

Fat 0.5

Sarsaparilla Syrup

Preparation Time: 15 minutes

Cooking Time: 40 minutes

Servings: 4

Ingredients :

Date sugar, 1 c

Sassafras root, 1 tbsp.

Sarsaparilla root, 1 c

Water, 2 c

Directions:

1. Firstly add all of the Ingredients to a mason jar. Screw on the lid, tightly, and shake everything together. Heat a water bath up to 160. Sit the mason jar into the water bath and allow it to infuse for about 40 minutes.

2. When the infusion time is almost up, set up an ice bath. Add half and half water and ice to a bowl. Carefully take the mason jar out of the water bath and place it into he ice bath. Allow it to sit in the ice bath for 15 to 20 minutes.

3. Strain the infusion out and into another clean jar.

Nutrition:

Calories 37

Sugar 2g

Protein 0.4g

Fat 0.3

Dandelion "Coffee"

Preparation Time: 15 minutes

Cooking Time: 10 minutes

Servings: 4

Ingredients :

• Nettle leaf, a pinch

• Roasted dandelion root, 1 tbsp.

• Water, 24 oz.

Directions:

1. To start, we will roast the dandelion root to help bring out its flavors. Feel free to use raw dandelion root if you want to, but roasted root brings out an earthy and complex flavor, which is perfect for cool mornings.

2. Simply add the dandelion root to a pre-warmed cast iron skillet. Allow the pieces to roast on medium heat until they start to darken in color, and you start to smell their rich aroma. Make sure that you don't let them burn because this will ruin your teas taste.

3. As the root is roasting, have the water in a pot and allow it to come up to a full, rapid boil. Once your dandelion is roasted, add it to the boiling water with the nettle leaf. Steep this for ten minutes.

4. Strain. You can flavor your tea with some agave if you want to. Enjoy.

Nutrition:

Calories 43

Sugar 1g

Protein 0.2g

Fat 0.3

Chamomile Delight

Preparation Time: 5 minutes

Cooking Time: 10 minutes

Servings: 3

Ingredients :

• Date sugar, 1 tbsp.

• Walnut milk, .5 c

• Alkaline Nerve/Stress Relief Herbal Tea, .25 c

• Burro banana, 1

Directions:

1. Prepare the tea according to the package Directions. Set to the side and allow to cool.

2. Once the tea is cooled, add it along with the above Ingredients to a blender and process until creamy and smooth.

Nutrition:

Calories 21

Sugar 0.8g

Protein 1.0g

Fat 0.2g

Cleanse Tea

Preparation Time: 10 minutes

Cooking Time: 5 minutes

Servings: 2

Ingredients :

• Blue Vervain

• Bladder wrack

• Irish Sea Moss

Directions:

1. Add the sea moss to your blender. This would be best as a gel. Just make sure that it is totally dry.

2. Place equal parts of the bladder wrack to the blender. Again this would be best as a gel. Just make sure that it is totally dry. To get the best results you need to chop these by hand.

3. Add equal parts of the blue vervain to the blender. You can use the roots to increase your iron intake and Nutritional healing values.

4. Process the herbs until they form a powder. This can take up to three minutes.

5. Place the powder into a non-metal pot and put it on the stove. Fill the pot half full of water. Make sure the herbs are totally immersed in water. Turn on the heat and let the liquid boil. Don't let it boil more than five minutes.

6. Carefully strain out the herbs. You can save these for later use in other recipes.

7. You can add in some agave nectar, date sugar, or key lime juice for added flavor.

Nutrition:

Calories 36

Sugar 6g

Protein 0.7g

Fat 0.3g

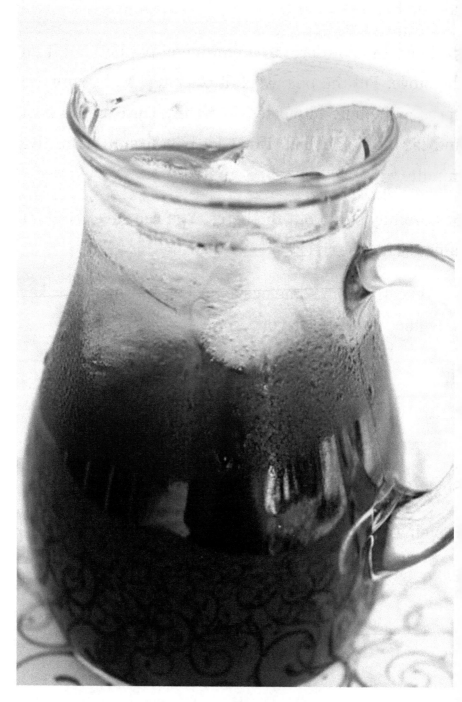

Immune Tea

Preparation Time: 10 minutes

Cooking Time: 20 minutes

Servings: 1

Ingredients :

• Echinacea, 1 part

• Astragalus, 1 part

• Rosehip, 1 part

• Chamomile, 1 part

• Elderflowers, 1 part

• Elderberries, 1 part

Directions:

1. Mix the herbs together and place them inside an airtight container.

2. When you are ready to make a cup of tea, place one teaspoon into a tea ball or bag, and put it in eight ounces of boiling water. Let this sit for 20 minutes.

Nutrition:

Calories 39

Sugar 1g

Protein 2g

Fat 0.6g

Ginger Turmeric Tea

Preparation Time: 5 minutes

Cooking Time: 15 minutes

Servings: 2

Ingredients :

• Juice of one key lime

• Turmeric finger, couple of slices

• Ginger root, couple of slices

• Water, 3 c

Directions:

1. Pour the water into a pot and let it boil. Remove from heat and put the turmeric and ginger in. Stir well. Place lid on pot and let it sit 15 minutes.

2. While you are waiting on your tea to finish steeping, juice one key lime, and divide between two mugs.

3. Once the tea is ready, remove the turmeric and ginger and pour the tea into mugs and enjoy. If you want your tea a bit sweet, add some agave syrup or date sugar.

Nutrition:

Calories 27

Sugar 5g

Protein 3g

Fat 1.0g

Relax Tea

Preparation Time: 5 minutes
Cooking Time: 10 minutes
Servings: 2

Ingredients :

• Rose petals, 2 parts

• Lemongrass, 2 parts

• Chamomile, 4 parts

Directions:

1. Pour all the herbs into a glass jar and shake well to mix.

2. When you are ready to make a cup of tea, add one teaspoon of the mixture for every serving to a tea strainer, ball, or bag. Cover with water that has boiled and let it sit for ten minutes.

3. If you like a little sweetness in your tea, you can add some agave syrup or date sugar.

Nutrition:

Calories 35

Sugar 3.4g

Protein 2.3g

Fat 1.5g

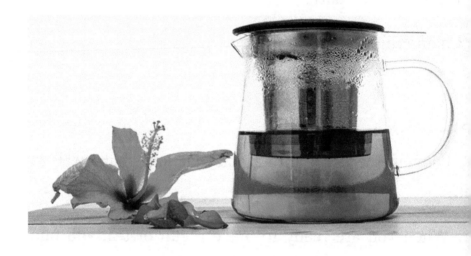

Lightning Source UK Ltd.
Milton Keynes UK
UKHW020702200521
384048UK00001B/19